YOUR KNOWLEDGE HAS VALUE

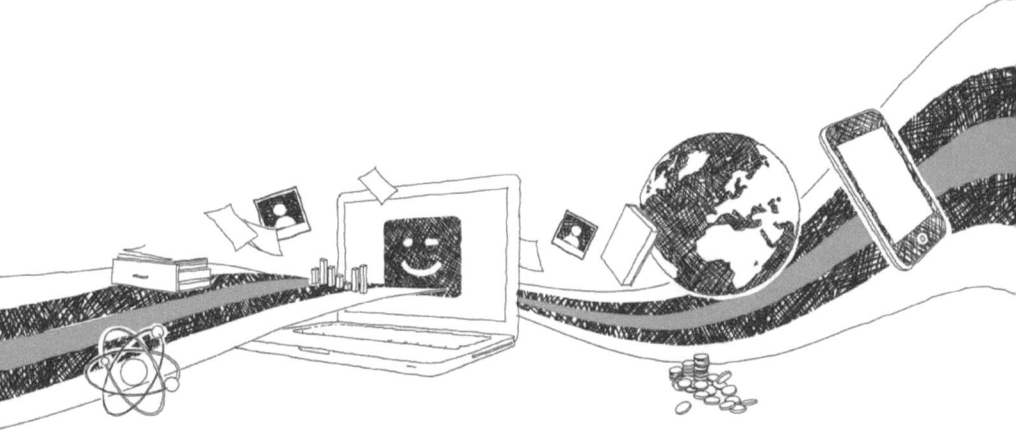

- We will publish your bachelor's and
  master's thesis, essays and papers

- Your own eBook and book -
  sold worldwide in all relevant shops

- Earn money with each sale

Upload your text at www.GRIN.com
and publish for free

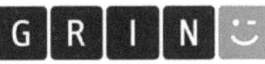

Bibliographic information published by the German National Library:

The German National Library lists this publication in the National Bibliography; detailed bibliographic data are available on the Internet at http://dnb.dnb.de .

This book is copyright material and must not be copied, reproduced, transferred, distributed, leased, licensed or publicly performed or used in any way except as specifically permitted in writing by the publishers, as allowed under the terms and conditions under which it was purchased or as strictly permitted by applicable copyright law. Any unauthorized distribution or use of this text may be a direct infringement of the author s and publisher s rights and those responsible may be liable in law accordingly.

Imprint:

Copyright © 2012 GRIN Verlag, Open Publishing GmbH
Print and binding: Books on Demand GmbH, Norderstedt Germany
ISBN: 9783656452232

This book at GRIN:

http://www.grin.com/en/e-book/229425/capstone-neglected-tropical-diseases-2

Donna Carrillo Lopez

Capstone - Neglected Tropical Diseases 2

Neglected Populations, NTDs and neglected symptoms

GRIN Publishing

GRIN - Your knowledge has value

Since its foundation in 1998, GRIN has specialized in publishing academic texts by students, college teachers and other academics as e-book and printed book. The website www.grin.com is an ideal platform for presenting term papers, final papers, scientific essays, dissertations and specialist books.

Visit us on the internet:

http://www.grin.com/

http://www.facebook.com/grincom

http://www.twitter.com/grin_com

Neglected Symptoms of Neglected Tropical Diseases
Challenges of advancing care in sub-Saharan Africa

Donna Carrillo Lopez, RN

Table of Contents

Introduction

In the year 2012, the world's population stands at 7 billion; out of this 7 billion, 1.4 billion live in extreme poverty, subsisting on less than $1.25 per day.[1] According to the United Nations' International Fund for Agricultural Development, 70% of the developing world's extreme poor population still lives in rural areas, with nearly a third living in sub-Saharan Africa (SSA).[2] SSA is a region that Oxfam depicts as a hurdler's race, in which "the weakest athletes face the highest hurdles."[3] In sub-Saharan Africa, life expectancy is thirty years less than the United States; the rural sector severely lacks social infrastructure including clean water, food, job opportunities, and housing. Basic healthcare is plagued by a dearth of access to transportation, resources, and healthcare professionals.[4] Within this climate and as a symptom of entrenched rural poverty, infectious diseases have become endemic to the region, affecting more than 500 million in rural sub-Saharan Africa.[5] The proliferation and persistence of infectious diseases disproportionately affect rural sub-Saharan Africa and stand as a hallmark for the neglect of poverty in rural areas. While the eradication of these diseases is now an international policy objective and a global health pledge by Bill Gates and the WHO, there remains a need to alleviate the pain and human suffering associated with these diseases, and to support the development of infrastructure that will empower vulnerable populations.

Following the HIV/AIDS pandemic and the emergence of novel infectious diseases, many of which occurred in sub-Saharan Africa, global attention has turned to neglected tropical diseases

---

[1] "We Can End Poverty 2015, The Millennium Development Goals." United Nations. http://www.un.org/millenniumgoals. 3 Mar 2012.
[2] United Nations International Fund for Agricultural Development. The Rural Poverty Report 2011. http://www.ifad.org/rpr2011/report/e/overview.pdf
[3] "Who We Are and Might Be: In Global Health, Excellence Demands Equity." *American Journal of Kidney Diseases.* Vol. 51, Iss. 1, Pages 145-154. Jan 2008.
[4] O'Neill, Edward. "Who We Are and Might Be: In Global Heath, Excellence Demands Equity. *American Journal of Kidney Diseases,* Volume 51, Issue 1.
[5] Hotez, PJ and A Kamath. "Neglected tropical diseases in sub-Saharan Africa: review of their prevalence, distribution, and disease burden." *PLoS Neglected Tropical Diseases.* 5 Aug 2009.

(NTDs). NTDs are a diverse group of infectious diseases with symptoms that are extremely debilitating and disfiguring; the "neglect" of these diseases is characterized by a notable dearth of research, development, and interventions to address their prevention and treatment.[6] NTDs are caused by pathogens that thrive in hot, humid environments and in areas where vectors are prevalent. These pathogens find a haven in the subtropical region of SSA, where intense poverty leaves populations vulnerable to a lack of access to clean water, adequate nutrition, housing, transportation, electricity, and primary healthcare.[7] NTDs are most prevalent among the 500 million people classified as the extreme poor in sub-Saharan Africa, who live on less than $1.25 a day; in SSA, they carry a burden of disease of more than 56.6 million Disability Adjusted Life Years (DALYs).[8] Peter Hotez, a global health expert and advocate, states that this burden is "equivalent to up to one-half of SSA's malaria disease burden and more than double that caused by tuberculosis…the overall burden of Africa's NTDs may be severely underestimated."[9] Research shows that no other continent in the world carries a burden of infectious disease equal in scope to the African continent.[10]

Recently, there has been a shift in the world's approach to fighting poverty and global health issues in low- and middle-income countries. NTDs are now accorded increasing attention. This concern for the increase in infectious diseases is manifested in an ambitious push by the Millennium Development Goals, which classify NTDs as a strategic priority, and in ongoing projects by the World Bank to address the economic impact of disease in debtor nations. These infectious diseases represent not only an issue of global health but also the deeply entrenched trends of inequality and

---

[6] Jamison, DT, JG Breman, AR Measham. *Priorities in Health.* World Bank: Washington DC, 2006.
[7] Manderson, L, J Aagaard, P Allotey, et al. *Social Research on Neglected Diseases of Poverty.* PLoS Negl Trop Dis. 3(2):e332. Global Climate Change for Africa Project 1998. 24 Feb 2009.
http://www.worldwildlife.org/bsp/bcn/learning/african/gcc1.htm
[8] Boutayeb, A. *Developing countries and neglected diseases: challenges and perspectives.* International Journal for Equity and Health. 2007.
[9] Hotez, PJ and A Kamath. *Neglected Tropical Diseases in Sub-Saharan Africa: Review of Their Prevalence, Distribution, and Disease Burden.* PLoS Negl Trop Dis 3(8):e412. 25 Aug 2009.
[10] Ibid.

neglect of populations; in the poor, rural areas of developing countries, these diseases become part of and perpetuate a cycle of poverty for individuals, families, and communities.

The increasing global focus on the health of the world's most impoverished populations also extends to human rights organizations, advocacy groups, and academic institutions. This has resulted in an abundance of journal articles, scholarly discussions, and global forums on the impact of infectious diseases in developing countries, as well as a growing number of non-governmental organizations (NGOs) devoted to reduce the prevalence of poverty and disease in poor countries.

The impetus to solve the growing problem of endemic infectious diseases has brought large investments from American and British aid agencies and organizations to fund the production of chemotherapeutic agents to combat these diseases. These investments are coordinated by pharmaceutical corporations such as GlaxoSmithKline, who donate over a billion treatments per year.[11] One example includes the $750 million investment for chemoprevention and treatment, which was recently given by the Gates Foundation to the Global Fund to Fight Aids, Tuberculosis and Malaria. This approach to mitigate the problem through funding and administration of chemical drugs has been challenged by recent concerns of field experts: according to an article in The Economist, "Bruno Gryseels of the Institute of Tropical Medicine in Antwerp fears that blanketing regions with medicines will make bugs drug-resistant."[12] While addressing short-term treatment needs is important to minimize the impact of infectious diseases, solving the long-term issues of global health requires the creation of sustainable solutions and a more collaborative process.

With the increased global attention and investments in chemical prevention, the subject of NTDs has not been neglected in recent years; however, the neglect of populations suffering

---

[11] "Neglected Tropical Diseases Hot Topic – the world's nastiest illnesses get some belated attention." *The Economist.* 4 Feb 2012.
[12] Ibid.

disproportionately from these diseases and the structural issues that hinder environmental prevention have persisted. The focus of investment and international organizations on chemical treatment as a solution to issues of global health and particularly epidemic infectious diseases ignores the historic memory of the economic development in the West during the age of industrialization. Surveillance of diseases was critical in the development of early public health measures. The measures envisioned by Florence Nightingale and implemented by Dr. John Snow during the cholera outbreak in London during the 1880s formed a foundation to address environmental prevention as a primary component of healthcare. Adequate supplies of safe and potable water, enriched food sources, functional transportation and energy infrastructure, and access to basic healthcare became the sine qua non for population health; only once these elements were addressed were vaccines and chemoprophylaxis introduced for prevention and treatment.

This paper will specifically address three NTDs whose pervasiveness and impact represent a metaphor for neglect: lymphatic filariasis, Buruli ulcer, and leprosy. In addition to investigating the impact of these three diseases and the general nature of NTDs, this paper will also explore the capacity of sub-Saharan Africa and the international community to address structural issues that hinder prevention and treatment.

Neglected Tropical Diseases

Definition

The World Health Organization (WHO) defines neglected tropical diseases (NTDs) as "hidden" diseases, as they affect almost exclusively extremely poor populations living in tropical rural areas beyond the reach of health services.[13] They comprise a diverse collection of primarily infectious diseases that thrive in the heat and humidity of tropical and sub-tropical climates. NTDs

---

[13] "Working to overcome the global impact of neglected tropical diseases: First WHO Report on Neglected Tropical Diseases." World Health Organization. 2010.

can have viral, protozoal, fungal, bacterial or filarial origins, and may be spread by insect or animal vectors – including mosquitoes, blackflies, snails, sandflies, and tsetse flies – or by contaminated water and soil infested with the eggs of worms. Their symptoms affect skin, nerves, lymphatic and subcutaneous tissue, causing lifelong, painful and disabling damage. They can also have an insidious onset, with severe impairments erupting after years of silent, subclinical infection.

The portfolio of WHO-targeted NTDs includes leishmaniasis, trypanosomiasis, Chagas, schistosomiasis, lymphatic filariasis, onchocerciasis, dracunculiasis, STHD, Leprosy, Buruli ulcer disease, trachoma, food borne trematode infection, cholera and yellow fever. While there are many more NTDs beyond the WHO focus, these diseases affect the particularly neglected populations suffering from NTDs. The WHO treats neglected tropical diseases as a group for two reasons. First, though medically diverse in terms of their causes and physical effects, all of these diseases cause severe disability and life-long impairments. Second, they are associated with conditions of poverty and tend to overlap geographically: NTDs proliferate in areas where clean water is scarce, sanitation is poor, housing is substandard, and disease-carrying insects are omnipresent. Grouping these diseases is also important for control programs, as many people are simultaneously infected with two or more diseases. Recent reports have suggested that as a group, NTDs have begun to approach the human and economic costs of malaria and tuberculosis in sub-Saharan Africa.[14]

'Neglected' diseases are characterized by a lack of effective, affordable, and accessible treatment as well as a low priority status for policy at international, domestic, or local levels. Neglected tropical diseases face a dearth of pharmacological research and development because they affect primarily poor populations in poor countries, with little impact on western societies. An

---

[14] Guerrant, RL Walker, DH., 1943, Weller, P. F. (2011) Tropical Infectious Disease: Principals, Pathogens and Practice; Elsevier: Chapter 11:71-75

estimated 500,000 to 1 million deaths occur as a result of NTDs each year;[15] nonetheless, because they are known for high morbidity and not high mortality, NTDs become invisible behind the 'big three' diseases that have prompted the most funding in Africa: HIV/AIDS, TB, and malaria.

With the world's rural poor encompassing the vast majority of the affected population, there is a direct link between poverty and NTDs, evidenced by a lack of basic infrastructure leaving these populations vulnerable to pathogens and without access to care. These diseases furthermore severely impact the already precarious health of poor populations and obstruct domestic development in low- and middle-income countries.

Impact of NTDs

NTDs not only impact the physical well being of those affected, but also create severe social and economic burdens in resource-limited countries beset with multiple epidemics. By curtailing human potential, NTDs anchor millions of poor people in poverty. The diminished economic productivity of young adults affected by these diseases causes an enormous burden, particularly among rural populations dependent on subsistence farming. NTDs also impair childhood growth and cognitive development, contracting opportunities for new generations to escape poverty.

Many of these diseases, particularly Buruli ulcer, leprosy, and lymphatic filariasis, are known to disable and deform, and because disease progression is often insidious, patients are often unaware of the need to seek care. During the progression of these diseases, infectious agents multiply, migrate through the body, and accumulate often silently in tissues, internal organs, or the lymphatic system until their symptoms take over and patients become disabled and disfigured. If not detected and treated in time, the damage they cause is irreversible. With the conspicuous, disfiguring symptoms of NTDs, individuals suffering from these diseases face not only pain and disability but also stigmatization and discrimination in their communities.

---

[15] "Neglected Tropical Diseases (NTDs)." Malaria Consortium.
http://www.malariaconsortium.org/pages/neglected_tropical_diseases.htm

The link between neglected tropical diseases and poverty is so strong that the prevalence of these diseases can serve as a proxy indicator of a country's socioeconomic development. Infectious diseases are the world's leading cause of premature deaths, causing 45% of deaths in low income countries and up to 63% of deaths in children under 4 years of age worldwide.[16] The World Health Organization estimates that approximately 1 billion people, or about one-seventh of the world's population, suffer from one or more neglected tropical diseases.[17]

Characterization of "Neglect"

With lower chronicity and mortality in comparison with the high-profile, highly fatal 'big three' diseases, NTDs have been designated to a low priority status in terms of research funding, development, and interventions. The facts presented by the Center for Disease Control depict the extremely detrimental costs of NTDs:

- 100% of low-income countries are affected by at least 5 neglected tropical diseases
- Worldwide, 149 countries and territories are affected by at least one NTD
- NTDs kill an estimated 534,000 people worldwide each year
- NTDs are a major cause of disease burden, resulting in approximately 57 million years of life lost due to premature disability and death
- Individuals are often afflicted with more than one NTD
- Tax costs for most NTD MDA programs is less than US $.50 per person per year[18]

Focus: Buruli Ulcer, Lymphatic Filariasis, Leprosy

Buruli ulcer, leprosy, and lymphatic filariasis are diseases of rural poverty; they are endemic in regions where water is unsafe to drink, personal hygiene is absent, sanitation is poor, housing is sub-standard, and disease vectors are omnipresent. All three diseases carry a burden of pain and

---

16 Environmental Health Perspectives. 2007 June; 115(6): A316–A317
17 WHO Fact Sheet No. 360. World Health Organization.
www.who.int/mediacentre/factsheets/fs360/en/index.htm.
18 "Neglected Tropical Diseases: Fast Facts." Centers for Disease Control and Prevention. 6 Jun 2011.
http://www.cdc.gov/globalhealth/ntd/fastfacts.html

9

suffering that is exacerbated by stigma and discrimination. The suffering is further compounded by the economic marginalization of victims, who are often disabled and unable to contribute as a valuable member of the community. Additionally, many of those who contract these diseases have co-endemic infectious diseases, including other NTDs.[19]

These three diseases are commonly given late treatment and are misdiagnosed by both traditional healers and allopathic physicians. As these diseases are epidemic in regions where healthcare professionals are already scarce due to a shortage of resources, these issues of diagnosis are extremely critical. In rural sub-Saharan Africa, the causes of late treatment include not only deficient healthcare infrastructure but also a critical lack of transportation that constitute a serious obstacle for patients who might seek treatment.

When an untreated or inadequately treated disease results in disfigurement and disability, this in turn creates further obstacles in seeking care. The odor or disfigurement is an intense source of embarrassment for those individuals who are relegated by circumstance to late treatment; malodorous infected Buruli ulcers, lymphedematous swollen legs, grossly swollen testicles, or facial disfigurement from lepromatous lesions may prevent individuals from leaving their dwelling, let alone travelling far to seek care. Within affected populations, there are certain groups that are particularly affected by social factors; because of their compromised social status in most rural sub-Saharan communities, women, children and minorities tend to experience greater suffering and stigmatization than men. These three diseases – Buruli ulcer, leprosy, and lymphatic filariasis – depict the extreme suffering endured by victims of NTDs and the impact of neglect on impoverished populations of sub-Saharan Africa.

---

[19] Hotez, Peter. "Devastating Global Impact of Neglected Tropical Diseases." Microbe Magazine. Aug 2009.

Buruli Ulcer

Buruli ulcer (BU) is a re-emerging disease that has been known by SSA traditional healers for decades, and is the third most prevalent mycobacterial disease after tuberculosis and leprosy.[20] BU has the highest endemic incidence in Cote d'Ivoire and Ghana, is spreading rapidly throughout western and central Africa, and is now present in over 33 countries. Its agent is mycobacterial ulcerans, which contains a unique toxic enzyme, called mycolactone, that is not characteristic of other mycobacteria. It is this enzyme that is responsible for nerve damage, which can cause the ulcer to be relatively painless until secondary infection or edema ensues.[21] The enzyme also causes massive tissue destruction, including the proliferation and metastases characteristic of later stages of this 'flesh-eating' disease. Early diagnosis of the disease and antibiotic therapy prevent dissemination, disfigurement, and long hospitalizations. Treatments recommended by the WHO include the following protocols:

1. Rifampicin and Streptomycin for 8 weeks as a first-line treatment for all forms of BU
   a. Nodular/uncomplicated cases treated without hospitalization
2. Surgery to remove necrotic tissue, cover skin defects and correct deformities
3. Interventions to prevent disabilities.[22]

Leprosy

Leprosy is a highly endemic disease present in many areas of developing countries. This disease is caused by a mycobacterium, M. leprae, which is an acid-fast bacillus of low-grade infectivity with a preference for cooler temperatures in body parts. With leprosy, the clinical reaction of infected patients depends on their immune response. If the cellular immune response is strong, the corresponding bacterial count will be low, and the patient will develop paucibacillary (PB) leprosy. If the cellular immune response is weak, the corresponding bacterial count will be

---

[20] Paul D. R. Johnson et. al. "Buruli Ulcer (M. ulcerans Infection): New Insights, New Hope for Disease Control." PLoS Medicine. 26 Apr 2005.
[21] Ibid.
[22] "Buruli Ulcer Treatment Recommendations." World Health Organization. http://www.who.int/Buruli/en

high, and the patient will develop multibacillary (MB) leprosy (more than 5 lesions). The type of leprosy dictates treatment regimen and determines pattern of systemic complications. The WHO recommends a multiple drug combination of rifampicin, clofazimine and dapsone for MB leprosy patients and rifampicin and dapsone for PB leprosy, emphasizing the importance of rifampicin, which is included in both forms of the disease.[23]

The disease pathogen is transmitted from individual to individual through nasal secretions and has an incubation period of two to five years. The disease is characterized by direct infection of the skin and nerves with associated immunological damage, and nerve involvement is responsible for repeated ulceration and paralysis affecting hands, feet and eyes. Lesions may result in severe deformity and, as a result, sufferers are often stigmatized and ostracized in their communities. This social stigma is an important cause of disability and places a high socioeconomic burden on the individual, their family and society. The persistence of leprosy as an epidemic infectious disease is often overlooked and neglected; it is estimated that the incidence is now 5.5 million worldwide. While it is difficult to estimate true prevalence, it is important for healthcare providers and communities to be aware of the disease for purposes of diagnosis: "leprosy should be considered whenever confronted by a chronic and symptomless skin rash that does not correspond with a common dermatosis or which does not respond to standard treatment for similar lesions."[24]

Lymphatic Filariasis

Lymphatic Filariasis (LF), also known as elephantiasis, is one of the most intensely stigmatizing and disfiguring neglected tropical diseases.[25] LF has one of the highest rates of disability of the NTDs and often generates profound pain in chronically ill patients. Pain in late infection is worsened by fungal and bacterial infections in affected areas, especially the limbs and

[23] "Leprosy Elimination." World Health Organization. http://www.who.int/lep/mdt/en/index.html. 9 Mar 2012.
[24] Zumla, Alimuddin and Gordon C. Cook. *Manson's Tropical Diseases*. 22nd Ed. London: Saunders, 2008.
[25] Chandy, A, A Thakur, and MP Singh. "A review of neglected tropical diseases: filariasis." *Asian Pacific Journal of Tropical Medicine*. 2011. 561-586.

genitals. Infection is usually acquired in childhood, but the painful and profoundly disfiguring visible manifestations of the disease typically occur later in life. 30% of 1.3 billion people affected by LF are the impoverished rural populations in SSA.[26]

Lymphatic filariasis is a lymphatic infection with a vector-born tissue dwelling nematode called filariae filariasis. It is transmitted by anopheles mosquitoes in sub-Saharan Africa. Depending on the species, adult filariae live in the lymphatics, blood vessels, skin, or connective tissues. Females produce larvae (microfilariae), which live in the bloodstream or skin. LF is confined to warm climates, as high temperature is necessary for parasites to develop in the vectors. The disease is also associated with poverty and environmental conditions that increase mosquito breeding, such as open sewage and stagnant pools of water. Microfilariae appear in the blood after a minimum of 8 months in one form of the disease called W. bancrofti, and 3 months in another form called B. malayi. The adult worms may live and produce microfilariae for more than 20 years, but on average the lifespan is shorter. Microfilariae have a lifespan of approximately 1 year and their density may reach 10,000 per ml of blood or more.[27]

Because lymphatic filariasis infection acquired in childhood is often asymptomatic, unnoticed lymphatic damage progressively occurs, with 40% of those affected having proteinuria and hematuria demonstrating renal involvement.[28] Currently, more than 1.3 billion people living in 81 countries are at risk.[29] Approximately 65% of those infected live in Southeast Asia, 30% in the African region, and the remainder in other tropical areas.[30] Lymphatic filariasis afflicts over 25 million men with genital disease and over 15 million people with lymphoedema.[31] Since the

---

[26] "Lymphatic Filariasis." World Health Organization. http://www.who.int/tdr/diseases-topics/lymphatic-filariasis/en. 9 Mar 2012.
[27] Ibid.
[28] Ibid.
[29] "Lymphatic Filariasis, Fact sheet N°102." World Health Organization. 2011.
http://www.who.int/mediacentre/factsheets/fs102/en
[30] Ibid.
[31] Ibid.

prevalence and intensity of infection are linked to poverty, its elimination is important not only for achieving the United Nations Millennium Development Goals but also in preventing the costly disability that worsens poverty and increases social marginalization.[32] Medications are used to prevent the transmission of the infection, and include anti-filarial drug combinations of either diethyl-carbamazine citrate (DEC) and albendazole or ivermecton and albendazole.[33]

Obstacles to Care and Factors that Facilitate the Spread of NTDs

There are several obstacles to care that are due to the intrinsic nature of these diseases. One of the main barriers to care of Buruli ulcer, leprosy and lymphatic filariasis is their asymptomatic nature in the early the stages of disease. Lymphatic filariasis, for example, is often diagnosed late, as chronic lymphoedema often doesn't manifest until early adulthood even if the disease is contracted during childhood. Buruli ulcer is also often diagnosed late, creating vulnerability to secondary infections. Resistance is another serious obstacle to care; leprosy's resistance to older drugs and treatments requires more advanced and expensive drugs, and while BU can be treated with a combination of antibiotic therapy, antibiotic resistance is on the horizon.

In addition to the nature of the diseases themselves, there are numerous social and structural factors that create obstacles to care and facilitate their spread. Mass drug administration and preventive chemotherapy have aimed and have succeeded to an extent at reducing current infections and preventing disability. Nonetheless, there are numerous social determinants that severely impede progress in addressing the needs of rural poor populations affected by NTDs:

- Lack of basic infrastructure: clean water, adequate nutrition, sanitation, housing, transportation, healthcare

---

[32] Ibid.
[33] "Lymphatic Filariasis." World Health Organization. http://www.who.int/tdr/diseases-topics/lymphatic-filariasis/en. 9 Mar 2012.

- o Half of the 1.8 million people residing in the northern region of Ghana lack access to safe drinking water[34]
- Dependence on donor aid, which diverts attention and resources away from local solutions
- Global funding for pharmaceuticals witnessed a $50 million drop from 2008 to 2009
    - o Leprosy, trachoma, and Buruli ulcer remained at the bottom of the funding scale, each receiving less than 0.3 % of global R&D investment[35]
- Inadequate number of health care practitioners in SSA
    - o In Uganda, there is one doctor for every 20,000 people and one traditional health practitioner per 200-400 people (36)
- Livelihoods rely on subsistence farming, which depends on unpredictable weather patterns

Prevention of Disease and Disability

Public Health Model: Levels of Prevention

The public health model designates three levels of prevention for disease: primary, secondary, and tertiary prevention. While the implementation of basic infrastructure and access to healthcare resources is fundamental to the development of preventive mechanisms in rural SSA, the elements of this model are equally important in addressing the prevention and treatment of NTDs.

Primary Prevention

Primary prevention focuses on community health prevention, utilizing the capacity of community leaders, traditional healers, teachers, and parents. It emphasizes proper hygiene, sanitation, and insect/vector spraying with insecticide, which addresses both malaria and LF. It also includes timely immunizations, protection of water, food supplies, prevention of trauma, and household improvements to prevent overcrowding.

---

[34] "Community Water Solutions: Our Work." http://www.communitywatersolutions.org/work.html
[35] Moran, Mary et. el. *Neglected Disease Research and Development: Is the Global Financial Crisis Changing R&D?* Policy Cures. Global Funding of Innovation for Neglected Diseases. Feb 2011.

Secondary Prevention

The main focus of secondary prevention is early diagnosis: to slow or block progression of disabilities and to increase the quality of life through early care of NTDs. Secondary prevention highlights the need for adequate infrastructure for rural people to access healthcare facilities. It is essential for individuals affected by these diseases to have access to these facilities in order to identify and treat their symptoms at an early stage of their illness.

Tertiary Prevention

The main aim of tertiary care is to slow or prevent the progression of a disability from NTDs through rehabilitation and care of pain. Prompt diagnosis and treatment are followed by rehabilitation and post-treatment recovery; patient education is also incorporated to avoid dramatic behavioral and lifestyle changes. Tertiary care targets social stigma by empowering those affected and preventing disability. In LF, for example, infection and acute attacks are prevented through hygiene and special massage techniques, and antibiotics are used for secondary infections. With leprosy, once the patient is on appropriate antibiotics, neuropathic pain is assessed and intervention is used to prevent physical and psychological morbidity (depression). For Buruli ulcer, contractures are prevented through guided movement, dressings, surgery, and antibiotics.[36]

Stigma is an additional concern of tertiary prevention. BU, LF, and leprosy have long incubation and latency periods. LF begins to manifest in extremity and genital swelling while BU manifests in ulceration with foul-smelling, weeping fluid. Leprosy is often diagnosed when disfigurement occurs with neuropathic pain. Disfigurement caused by these diseases results in isolation from normal social contacts and reluctance to travel and seek care. Prevalent religious, cultural beliefs that an affected person is cursed can ruin a family business and can perpetuate social

---

[36] Merrill, RM and TC Timmreck. *Introduction to Epidemiology, 4th ed.* London: Jones and Bartlett Publishers, 2006. 14-16.

marginalization. Stigma often results in worsening poverty and isolation from social networks and can impact an individual as severely as the physical manifestations of the disease.

Poverty and Infectious Diseases

The link between poverty and infectious diseases has been widely discussed in the field of global health; yet the extent to which poverty fuels a cycle of neglect of populations and the spread of disease is often grossly underestimated. Approximately 700 million people suffer from neglected tropical diseases. Of this population, 1 in 10 suffer from schistosomiasis, 1 in 20 from lymphatic filariasis and trachoma, and 1 in 50 suffer from onchocerciasis.[37] Additionally, one or more of the 7 most common NTDs – ascariasis, trichuriasis, hookworm, schistosomiasis, L.F. trachoma, and onchocerciasis – affect 1 billion people.[38]

Infrastructure deficits in rural areas of resource-poor countries include lack of access to clean water, extremely poor sanitation, inadequate diet causing micronutrient and caloric deficiencies, limited or no access to basic healthcare, overcrowded housing, and limited transportation.[39] These factors combine to create an environment in which the poor face an everyday struggle to simply remain healthy.

Environmental Factors

There are several reasons why NTDs disproportionately affect countries in sub-Saharan Africa. First, SSA countries have a heavy reliance on natural resources for survival and commonly lack financial and technical means to reduce vulnerability to climate change.[40] For the rural poor who rely on subsistence farming, environmental shocks such as droughts and floods can have severe

---

[37] Hotez, Peter. "Neglected Infections of Poverty Among the Indigenous People of the Arctic." PLoS. 26 Jan 2010. 4(1):e606
[38] Hotez, Peter. "Neglected Infections of Poverty Among the Indigenous People of the Arctic." PLoS. 26 Jan 2010. 4(1):e606
[39] Ibid.
[40] "Global Climate Change for Africa Project." *Biodiversity Support Program*. 1998. http://www.worldwildlife.org/bsp/bcn/learning/african/gcc1.htm. 11 Dec 2011

and long-lasting impacts on their livelihoods and health. With micronutrient and caloric deficits from a lack of nutrition, these populations often suffer severe immune deficiencies, which leave them particularly vulnerable to pathogens in their environment. A lack of basic infrastructure further compounds the effects of environmental vulnerability on the health of the rural population, limiting access to other sources of nourishment and basic care.

Limitations of Current Healthcare System

Deficient healthcare systems are a critical issue affecting the spread of disease in SSA. Most sub-Saharan countries have inadequate social infrastructure and government policies to promote the care of pain and effectively treat the symptoms of chronic infectious diseases, including NTDs. These countries lack a prioritized agenda to improve the efficiency and quality of care for rural populations, where few physicians are available or accessible. In Uganda, for example, there is one physician for every 19,000 people, one nurse for every 4,000, and one traditional healer for every 450.[41] While traditional healers fill the gap in accessible health care providers for 80 percent of the population, this care often delays timely medical diagnosis and treatment that could prevent progression and disability of the disease.

Stigmatization, Discrimination, and Cultural Barriers

Cultural beliefs represent another essential element of the disproportionate impact of NTDs in SSA. Stigma is defined as "a social process, experienced or anticipated, characterized by exclusion, rejection, blame, or devaluation."[42] It is a significant determinant of healthcare systems in SSA because serious diseases and chronic pain are regarded with superstition and fear in many areas. Common beliefs in SSA, especially in rural villages, regard those suffering from disfiguring

---

[41] Merriman, A and R Harding. "Pain Control in the African Context: the Ugandan introduction of affordable morphine to relieve suffering at the end of life." Philosophy, Ethics, and Humanities in Medicine. 8 Jul 2010. 4-10.
[42] Person, B, LK Bartholomew, M Gypong, et al. "Health related stigma among women with lymphatic filariasis from the Dominican Republic and Ghana." Social Science and Medicine. Nov 2008. 68:30-38

and disabling diseases as bewitched or plagued by malignant supernatural forces.[43] The discrimination that affected individuals face has huge implications for their social and economic status. Stigma marginalizes affected populations, creating a worsening cycle of poverty which itself increases vulnerability of contracting disease, particularly neglected tropical diseases.

While there is no Swahili word for lymphatic filariasis, there are words to convey the signs of infection, including enlarged testicles, called *Mahusha*. However, this term has a strong association with sex, witchcraft, hernias, diet and sickness sent by God.[44] Much of the rural sub-Saharan population is unaware that LF is an infection caused by mosquitoes. *Matende* is the name for the swollen limbs of LF; this term is also attributed to witchcraft and to a fever known as *mgonza*. There is minimal association between the ingestion of drugs such as albendazole and ivermeectin and the alleviation of symptoms.[45] In fact, those who were asked to take the drugs often became suspicious, wondering if this was an "unspoken agenda by the government to decrease birth rates or experiment on the poor."[46] Buruli ulcer and leprosy are also diseases of stigma, facing strong beliefs in the community that the affected have been cursed or victims of witchcraft. This highlights the marginalization of victims that occurs with stigma and cultural belief systems.

International Policy and Neglect of Poverty

In the 1980s and 1990s, the World Bank and International Monetary Fund (IMF) engineered structural adjustment programs (SAPS), designed to stem the tide of loan defaults by debtor nations. Though they were intended to stabilize developing economies and reduce global poverty, the SAPs created severe cash flow deficits in economically besieged African countries. This reversal of monetary flows "caused millions of sub-Saharan Africans to go without education and health

---

[43] Ribera, JM, KP Grietens, E Toomer, et al. "A Word of Caution Against the Stigma Trend in Neglected Tropical Disease, Research and Control." PLoS Negl Trop Dis. Oct 2009. 3(10): e445
[44] Allen, T and M Parker. "The 'other diseases' of the Millennium Development Goals: rhetoric and reality of free drug distribution to cure the poor's parasites." Third World Quarterly. Vol. 32, No. 1, 2011. 91-117.
[45] Ibid.
[46] Ibid.

care."[47] These policies were aligned with a priority on fiscal balance and low inflation, but rather than reversing poverty they diminished resources and prevented investment in medical education. The consequences included a lack of medical supplies, resources, and trained physicians and nurses. With this lack of capacity, pain care in rural areas was relegated to traditional healers, and patients were left with little or no access to medications like morphine for relief of moderate to severe pain.

By the end of the 1990s, world leaders recognized that the diminishing health of global populations was not only worsening poverty but also affecting the development of low- and middle-income countries throughout the world. It became clear that the deteriorating health of the world's "bottom billion" had enormous implications for social, political, and economic stability as well as national security in developing countries. Thus, health was a pressing matter of global concern.

Implications for Pain Care in SSA and Recommendations for Future Action

During the 1980s, HIV/AIDS decimated young adult populations in SSA and around the world. Pain assessment was not included in the way that medical experts and healthcare professionals defined the disease and its treatment. With the emergence of anti-retroviral treatments, victims were able to live longer and experience the neuropathic pain common to the disease; thereby, pain became a factor in treatment of HIV/AIDS. In the West, the International Association for the Study of Pain (IASP) published in 1996 a 'call for action' for physicians to consider the under-treatment of pain in HIV/AIDS, a disease that followed the poor treatment of cancer pain in earlier decades.[48] Nine years later, Brennan, Carr and Cousins published an article declaring pain management an issue of human rights.[49] Patients living with chronic pain were found

---

[47] O'Neill, E. *Poverty, Structural Violence and Racism in a World Out of Balance.* Race and the Global Politics of Health Inequity. 2009. 115-138

[48] "Pain in AIDS: A Call for Action." Pain: Clinical Updates. *International Association for the Study of Pain.* Vol 4, Iss 1. Mar 1996.

[49] Brennan, F, DB Carr, and M Cousins. "Pain Management: A Fundamental Right." Anesthesia and Analgesia. Vol 105, No.1. Jul 2007.

to be associated with lower socioeconomic status, which was attributed to their pain-associated

disabilities. A deficient system of pain management further compromised the social, economic and

psychological well-being of this population:

> *In addition to cultural, medical and religious impediments, entrenched political and legal barriers discourage adequate pain management. Opioids remain the drugs of choice for the treatment of moderate to severe pain, regardless of etiology...In 2004 data published by the International Narcotics Control Board (INCB), 6 nations accounted for 79% of medical morphine consumption and 120 consumed little or none. Two principal impediments to opioid availability are restriction and cost.[50]*

As the IASP declared, "chronic pain is a major health care problem, a disease in its own right" and

those who live in pain do not suffer alone; societies that fail to create policies for the management

of pain suffer a loss of human capital and diminished social and economic well-being.[51]

Pain treatment in Africa as a whole is severely lacking mainly due to poor distribution

channels for medications and lack of funding. Treating pain in this context, however, does not

follow the traditional mechanical path. Effective pain management must involve a public

information campaign that educates local communities about the causes of the diseases and the

necessary care, collaboration between the private and public sectors, and prevention of disabilities.

It is estimated that 80% of the world's population has no access to prescribed pain relief.

This lack of pain care is an important consideration in evaluating the actual impact of chronic

infectious diseases, especially in extreme conditions. For example, the occurrence of Buruli ulcer

can cause patients to endure necessary amputation and profound disability when painful

contractures intensify. Pain care is also important in the care of leprosy, with neuropathic pain

often continuing long after treatment. The obstacles to establishing pain care in SSA include: "the

failure of many governments to put in place functioning drug supply systems; the failure to enact

policies on pain treatment and palliative care; poor training of healthcare workers; the existence of

---

[50] Ibid.
[51] "Unrelieved Pain Is A Major Global Healthcare Problem." *International Association for the Study of Pain.* www.iasp-pain.org

unnecessarily restrictive drug control regulations and practices; fear among healthcare workers of legal sanctions for legitimate medical practice; and the inflated cost of pain treatment."[52]

It is important to observe that pain treatment medications are not evenly distributed worldwide; approximately 89% of the total world consumption of morphine occurs in North America and Europe. Low and middle income countries consume only 6% of the morphine used worldwide, even though they are home to about half of all cancer patients and more than 90% of HIV infections.[53]

Pain Implications of 3 NTDs

The three NTDs discussed in this paper – Buruli ulcer, leprosy, and lymphatic filariasis – are characterized by chronic and severe acute pain. Although leprosy was formerly considered painless, clinicians now view it as the most common cause of painful mononeuritis. Buruli ulcer pain is often due to secondary infections, trapped nerves or surgical scar tissue, and inflammatory pain prior to and following antibiotic therapy. Lymphatic filariasis sufferers experience severe pain during secondary infections in acute attacks. With the lack of a robust pain management model and limited healthcare access in rural sub-Saharan Africa where these diseases are most prevalent, affected populations in this region suffer from more chronic pain conditions. There is thus an essential need for an innovative model of pain management in the SSA region.

Recommendations for Pain Management

In 1993, Dr. Anne Merriman founded Hospice Uganda as a model for palliative care in sub-Saharan Africa. Since that time, medical and nursing schools at Makerere University have incorporated training in palliative and pain care, utilizing available oral morphine.[54] Through her efforts in raising awareness, the Ministry of Health collaborated in facilitating the importation of

---

[52] Lohman, D, R Schleifer, and JJ Amon. "Access to pain treatment as a human right." BMC Medicine. 20 Jan 2010. 8:8
[53] Ibid.
[54] Merriman

morphine powder, using a formula created and perfected in Singapore during Dr. Merriman's tenure there as a physician.[55] Dr. Merriman pointed to the lack of affordable morphine for palliative care in African countries, and through her efforts catalyzed the development of palliative care programs throughout the region.[56] In her model, Dr. Merriman combined advocacy, training, education and community outreach and employed healthcare staff trained in identifying pain symptoms as well as administering oral morphine. In Uganda, the model was implemented with the help of Catholic charity hospitals.

Merriman stated recently that it was her hope that the institutional changes made in Uganda would also be adopted by other African countries to ensure humane treatment for people in pain beyond terminal care. Dr. Merriman recognized not only the burden of pain in terminal diseases but also the necessity to create lasting structural changes in Uganda to engage the government, the Ministry of Health, and policymakers. Through this collaborative process, Hospice Uganda was able to create the necessary community networks to sustain the care of pain while creating awareness of diseases and their treatment.

The holistic approach to pain care begins with the availability of morphine, the education and training of healthcare professionals in pain management, and a collaborative process involving community leaders and policymakers. Only through this approach can we alleviate the suffering and ensure the dignity of populations affected by these diseases.[57] Dr. Merriman's model provides an inspiration and a guide to diminish the impact of NTDs in sub-Saharan Africa.

Recommendations to Address Stigmatization and Discrimination
Social stigma associated with neglected tropical diseases are acute, especially among those known for their body disfigurement, such as Buruli ulcer, lymphatic filariasis and leprosy. With

---

[55] Ibid.
[56] Ibid.
[57] Merriman

23

minimal social infrastructure in rural areas, 'destigmatization' in societies relies on education through outreach from village chiefs, teachers, and other community leaders. This model of 'destigmatization' has been utilized in India to counter the stigma of leprosy, while educating the villagers on the bacterial causes and incorporating an awareness of multidrug therapy so that disfigurement can be avoided or controlled.[58]

Course of Action to Empower Affected Populations

The fight against neglected tropical diseases represents an opportunity to mitigate rural poverty in sub-Saharan Africa and in other continents where poverty is strongly associated with infectious disease. In this undertaking, history provides a guide to the future. Dr. John Snow's discovery of a single waterspout as the vector causing the cholera outbreak in London in the 1880s represented a breakthrough highlighting the necessity to reduce the environmental causes of pathogens. Today, this translates into the epidemiological model of infectious diseases; in rural sub-Saharan Africa, a lack of basic infrastructure places populations at high risk to contraction and spread of infectious diseases. Hence, there is a necessity to design a reliable infrastructure that provides clean water, sanitation, adequate housing, transportation, and access to basic healthcare in order to address basic prevention of these diseases.

The innovative nature of Hospice Uganda brought much needed change in the country's delivery of healthcare, and resulted in other African countries adopting more horizontal policies. This horizontal movement took root in its potential to empower people living in rural areas with a more precise understanding of the diseases, which counters superstitions and stigmas surrounding them. While disability care is not the central focus of this paper, it is worth noting that Dr. Merriman's model of empowering patients, villages, local chiefs, and governments can be the way forward in providing welfare to disabled patients and their families through outreach programs.

---

[58] Weiss, MG. *Stigma and the Social Burden of Neglected Tropical Diseases.* Vol 2/Issue5:e237. PLoS. May 2008.

Inclusion, education, and a sense of empowerment are the main attributes of this model, which is targeted toward the individuals most affected by disease and poverty.

Conclusion

The genesis of neglected tropical diseases lies in rural poverty. These diseases occur disproportionately in sub-Saharan Africa, where resource-poor areas are often ignored with urban-focused development agendas. The term "neglected" denotes the lack of research, development, and policy interventions to address the needs of affected populations, but also the structural neglect of the poor rural populations in these countries. Organizations, government agencies, and academic institutions now understand the need to harness efforts to cope with the impact and spread of NTDs from a public health perspective.

The WHO, PEPVAR, and other organizations are currently advancing efforts to include NTDs into the public health framework that is used to combat HIV/AIDS, tuberculosis and malaria – including primary, secondary, and tertiary prevention utilizing the epidemiological model as a framework. Primary prevention strategies to prevent these diseases must include not only vaccinations and chemoprophylaxis but also policy measures to address infrastructure deficits. This includes the provision of sustainable clean water, nutrient-enriched food, adequate housing, community health education, access to transportation, and healthcare provisions to enable early diagnosis and treatment. The impact of disease must be addressed by the early prevention of disabilities, community outreach to diminish social stigma, and empowerment of affected individuals and their families.

Anne Merriman's founding model of Hospice Uganda is uniquely suited to address the opiophobia, opioignorance, and low capacity of pain care in SSA. The hospice model offers great promise for not only end-of-life pain and suffering but also for the pain that accompanies the chronic stages of NTDs. This model may also help diminish the disabilities associated with chronic NTDs. This model is community-based and gains ownership through a multi-pronged approach – delivering change not only vertically through domestic policy change but also horizontally through pain management training for health care professionals and community involvement.

There is great hope for the mitigation and care of NTDs if there is a global, national, and local effort involving government entities and NGOs to design policies and incentives that break the intergenerational cycle of poverty. In addition to chemoprophylaxis (multi-drug administration), immunization, and investment, global health organizations should begin to place the empowerment of populations as a first priority. Anne Merriman's vision is the expansion of her hospice pain model into the care and treatment of chronic pain of NTDs across sub-Saharan Africa. This novel model of care has the potential to empower rural communities and pave the way for more effective and inclusive public health interventions.

Two cycles – neglect of populations and poverty – reinforce each other and perpetuate the spread of disease in rural areas. This paradigm has been demonstrated in the disproportionate impact of NTDs in rural sub-Saharan Africa, and presents the challenges Africa faces in properly tackling the spread of these diseases. History has shown that top-down approaches to healthcare have practical limitations in terms of addressing the complex, multifaceted determinants of these diseases. As Bill Gates observed at a meeting to endorse the London Declaration on Neglected Tropical Diseases in January 2012, as we advance toward sustainable solutions that incorporate these elements in the prevention and care of NTDs, it is our hope that "maybe as the decade goes on, people will wonder whether these should be called 'neglected' diseases."

Endnotes

1. "We Can End Poverty 2015, The Millennium Development Goals." United Nations. http://www.un.org/millenniumgoals. 3 Mar 2012.

2. United Nations International Fund for Agricultural Development. The Rural Poverty Report 2011. http://www.ifad.org/rpr2011/report/e/overview.pdf

3. "Who We Are and Might Be: In Global Health, Excellence Demands Equity." *American Journal of Kidney Diseases.* Vol. 51, Iss. 1, Pages 145-154. Jan 2008.

4. O'Neill, Edward. "Who We Are and Might Be: In Global Heath, Excellence Demands Equity. *American Journal of Kidney Diseases,* Volume 51, Issue 1.

5. Hotez, PJ and A Kamath. "Neglected tropical diseases in sub-Saharan Africa: review of their prevalence, distribution, and disease burden." *PLoS Neglected Tropical Diseases.* 5 Aug 2009.

6. Jamison, DT, JG Breman, AR Measham. *Priorities in Health.* World Bank: Washington DC, 2006.

7. Manderson, L, J Aagaard, P Allotey, et al. *Social Research on Neglected Diseases of Poverty.* PLoS Negl Trop Dis. 3(2):e332. Global Climate Change for Africa Project 1998. 24 Feb 2009. http://www.worldwildlife.org/bsp/bcn/learning/african/gcc1.htm

8. Boutayeb, A. *Developing countries and neglected diseases: challenges and perspectives.* International Journal for Equity and Health. 2007.

9. Hotez, PJ and A Kamath. *Neglected Tropical Diseases in Sub-Saharan Africa: Review of Their Prevalence, Distribution, and Disease Burden.* PLoS Negl Trop Dis 3(8):e412. 25 Aug 2009.

10. Ibid.

11. "Neglected Tropical Diseases Hot Topic – the world's nastiest illnesses get some belated attention." *The Economist.* 4 Feb 2012.

12. Ibid.

13. "Working to overcome the global impact of neglected tropical diseases: First WHO Report on Neglected Tropical Diseases." World Health Organization. 2010.

14. Guerrant, RL Walker, DH., 1943, Weller, P. F. (2011) Tropical Infectious Disease: Principals, Pathogens and Practice; Elsevier: Chapter 11:71-75

15. "Neglected Tropical Diseases (NTDs)." Malaria Consortium. http://www.malariaconsortium.org/pages/neglected_tropical_diseases.htm

16. Environmental Health Perspectives. 2007 June; 115(6): A316–A317

17. WHO Fact Sheet No. 360. World Health Organization. www.who.int/mediacentre/factsheets/fs360/en/index.htm.

18. "Neglected Tropical Diseases: Fast Facts." Centers for Disease Control and Prevention. 6 Jun 2011. http://www.cdc.gov/globalhealth/ntd/fastfacts.html

19. Hotez, Peter. "Devastating Global Impact of Neglected Tropical Diseases." Microbe Magazine. Aug 2009.

20. Paul D. R. Johnson et. al. "Buruli Ulcer (M. ulcerans Infection): New Insights, New Hope for Disease Control." PLoS Medicine. 26 Apr 2005.

21. Ibid.

22. "Buruli Ulcer Treatment Recommendations." World Health Organization. http://www.who.int/Buruli/en

23. "Leprosy Elimination." World Health Organization. http://www.who.int/lep/mdt/en/index.html. 9 Mar 2012.

24. Zumla, Alimuddin and Gordon C. Cook. *Manson's Tropical Diseases.* 22nd Ed. London: Saunders, 2008.

25. Chandy, A, A Thakur, and MP Singh. "A review of neglected tropical diseases: filariasis." *Asian Pacific Journal of Tropical Medicine.* 2011. 561-586.

26. "Lymphatic Filariasis." World Health Organization. http://www.who.int/tdr/diseases-topics/lymphatic-filariasis/en. 9 Mar 2012.

27. Ibid.

28. Ibid.

29. "Lymphatic Filariasis, Fact sheet N°102." World Health Organization. 2011. http://www.who.int/mediacentre/factsheets/fs102/en

30. Ibid.

31. Ibid.

32. Ibid.

33. "Lymphatic Filariasis." World Health Organization. http://www.who.int/tdr/diseases-topics/lymphatic-filariasis/en. 9 Mar 2012.

34. "Community Water Solutions: Our Work." http://www.communitywatersolutions.org/work.html

35. Moran, Mary et. el. *Neglected Disease Research and Development: Is the Global Financial Crisis Changing R&D?* Policy Cures. Global Funding of Innovation for Neglected Diseases. Feb 2011.

36. Merrill, RM and TC Timmreck. *Introduction to Epidemiology, 4th ed.* London: Jones and Bartlett Publishers, 2006. 14-16.

37. "Neglected Tropical Diseases." *The Future of Global Health: Ingredients for a Bold and Effective U.S. Initiative.* Vermont Global Health Coalition. Oct 2009. http://www.theglobalhealthinitiative.org/documents/report_ntd.pdf

38. Hotez, Peter. "Neglected Infections of Poverty Among the Indigenous People of the Arctic." PLoS. 26 Jan 2010. 4(1):e606

39. Ibid.

40. "Global Climate Change for Africa Project." *Biodiversity Support Program.* 1998. http://www.worldwildlife.org/bsp/bcn/learning/african/gcc1.htm. 11 Dec 2011

41. Merriman, A and R Harding. "Pain Control in the African Context: the Ugandan introduction of affordable morphine to relieve suffering at the end of life." Philosophy, Ethics, and Humanities in Medicine. 8 Jul 2010. 4-10.

42. Person, B, LK Bartholomew, M Gypong, et al. "Health related stigma among women with lymphatic filariasis from the Dominican Republic and Ghana." Social Science and Medicine. Nov 2008. 68:30-38

43. Ribera, JM, KP Grietens, E Toomer, et al. "A Word of Caution Against the Stigma Trend in Neglected Tropical Disease, Research and Control." PLoS Negl Trop Dis. Oct 2009. 3(10): e445

44. Allen, T and M Parker. "The 'other diseases' of the Millennium Development Goals: rhetoric and reality of free drug distribution to cure the poor's parasites." Third World Quarterly. Vol. 32, No. 1, 2011. 91-117.

45. Ibid.

46. Ibid.

47. O'Neill, E. *Poverty, Structural Violence and Racism in a World Out of Balance.* Race and the Global Politics of Health Inequity. 2009. 115-138

48. "Pain in AIDS: A Call for Action." Pain: Clinical Updates. *International Association for the Study of Pain.* Vol 4, Iss 1. Mar 1996.

49. Brennan, F, DB Carr, and M Cousins. "Pain Management: A Fundamental Right." Anesthesia and Analgesia. Vol 105, No.1. Jul 2007.

50. Ibid.

51. "Unrelieved Pain Is A Major Global Healthcare Problem." *International Association for the Study of Pain.* www.iasp-pain.org

52. Lohman, D, R Schleifer, and JJ Amon. "Access to pain treatment as a human right." BMC Medicine. 20 Jan 2010. 8:8

53. Ibid.

54. Merriman

55. Ibid.

56. Ibid.

57. Merriman

58. Weiss, MG. *Stigma and the Social Burden of Neglected Tropical Diseases.* Vol 2/Issue5:e237. PLoS. May 2008.

YOUR KNOWLEDGE HAS VALUE

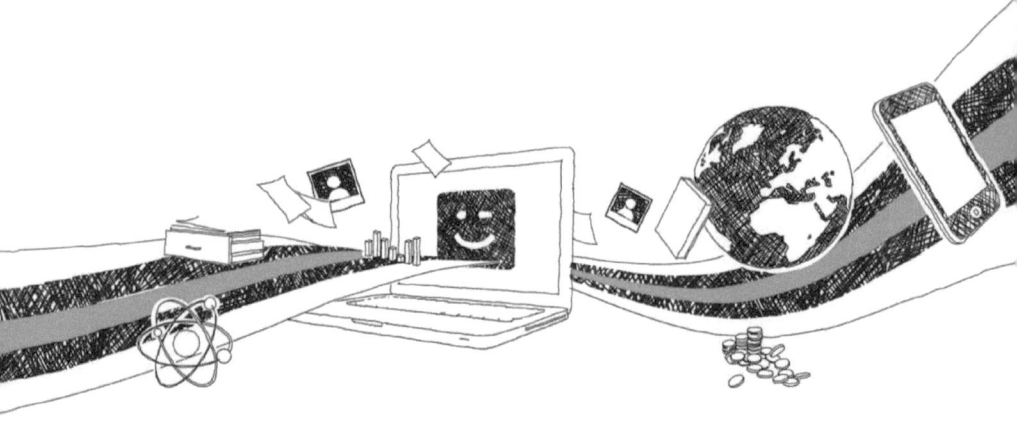

- We will publish your bachelor's and
  master's thesis, essays and papers

- Your own eBook and book -
  sold worldwide in all relevant shops

- Earn money with each sale

Upload your text at www.GRIN.com
and publish for free

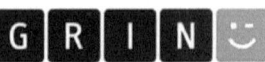